STRETCH
FOR
HEALTH

NO-NONSENSE HEALTH GUIDE

STRETCH FOR HEALTH

Easy-Does-It Exercises for a More Limber, Flexible Body

By the Editors of
Prevention® Magazine

Longmeadow Press

Notice

This book is intended as a reference volume only, not as a medical manual or guide to self-treatment. It is not intended as a substitute for the medical advice of physicians. The reader should regularly consult a physician in general, and particularly for any symptoms. If you suspect that you have a medical problem, we urge you to seek competent medical help. Keep in mind that exercise and nutritional needs vary from person to person, depending on age, sex, health status and individual variations. The information here is intended to help you make informative decisions about your health, not as a substitute for any treatment that may have been prescribed by your doctor.

Published April 1987 for Longmeadow Press, 201 High Ridge Road, Stamford, CT 06904. No part of this book may be reproduced or used in any form or by any means, electronic or mechanical, including photocopying, recording, or by any information storage and retrieval system, without permission in writing from the publisher.

Library of Congress Cataloging-in-Publication Data

Stretch for health.

    (No-nonsense health guide)
    1. Exercise.   2. Physical fitness.   3. Stretch (Physiology)   I. Prevention (Emmaus, Pa.)   II. Series.
GV505.S77   1987   613.7'1   87-4120
ISBN 0-681-40130-3   paperback

Special thanks to Jeff Meade for compiling and editing the information in this book.

Book design by Acey Lee and Lisa Gatti

Photographs by Margaret Skrovanek: pp. 58, 59, 61, 62, 63, 64, 68, 69, 70, 71, 72, 73, 74; Christie C. Tito: pp. 49, 50, 51, 52, 53, 54, 55.

Illustrations by Susan Rosenberger

2   4   6   8   10   9   7   5   3   1   paperback

Contents

Why Stretch?

Why is flexibility crucial to health? To understand, we first have to understand just what flexibility is. Scientists define it as the "range of motion about a joint"—the maximum degree to which you can reach, turn, twist, swing and bend.

In fact, many scientists believe that muscles deprived of exercise actually get shorter as we grow older. The more these muscles are neglected, the shorter they will get, which is why being flexible is so important to health. By staying flexible we stay supple, loose—and young.

What are some of the most important facts researchers have found out about flexibility and exercise over the years?

- First of all, stretching *does* improve flexibility. A study at the University of Oregon showed that women who did routine stretching exercises became significantly more limber. And those who were considered in "average" shape at the beginning of the semester-long experiment made the greatest gains.

- Warm-up exercises greatly improve mobility. Even a single preliminary movement—a Toe Touch, for example—results in a better score for that test. *Research Quarterly* reported a study involving 33 college men who were tested in the Toe Touch over a five-week period. Men who practiced the Toe Touch and other exercises before the test did considerably better than men who started cold. (However, as we explain in chapter 13, some people with low back problems should not do Toe Touches.)
- There is no such thing as "normal" flexibility. This is because the range of natural movement varies so greatly from person to person. You can admire the person who can touch his toes with his elbows, but you don't have to be able to do it to be in the same physical shape.
- Flexibility is not the same throughout the body. Flexibility in one joint doesn't guarantee equal range of motion in other body parts. So you have to loosen up *all* of you, not just your back or legs. This book will show you how.

How Flexible Are You?

How flexible are you? Well, get on your feet and we'll find out. The idea of this little test is to find out how easily you can bend your body without any strain or pain. But be careful! If you haven't bent over without bending your knees in ten years, or if you think it may aggravate a low back problem, don't force yourself. Here goes:

- Stand erect, with your hands at your sides and your feet together. Keeping your knees locked, bend slowly from the waist. Stop when you begin to feel a tight resistance in the back of your legs or in your back. Are your fingers dangling somewhere around your knees? If so, you could use a little practice. Flexible men have no problem touching their toes. And women can even rest their palms on the floor.

- Now sit on the floor with your legs stretched out in front of you. Put an eight-inch-high book upright between your knees. Clasp your hands behind your head. Keeping your legs flat, lean forward until you feel that telltale strain. The really

1

flexible person can touch the book with his forehead.

- Lie flat on your stomach with your hands clasped behind your neck and your feet touching the floor. How far can you raise your chin off the floor without straining? Don't be surprised if you can't raise it at all. The truly flexible person can get from 12 to 18 inches off the floor.

Take this test again after you've read this book and practiced some of the stretching routines for a few weeks. You'll probably be proud of your progress.

Four Rules for Safer Stretching

To stretch or not to stretch?

This question has been a bone of contention ever since a survey done several years ago showed that marathon runners who were regular stretchers suffered *more* injuries than runners who didn't stretch at all. Could we be literally pulling ourselves apart at the seams with our well-intended efforts to be more limber?

The National Strength and Conditioning Association (NSCA) posed that question to six top experts in the sportsmedicine field, and some very good advice emerged.

Advice from the Experts

One point the experts are adamant about is when to stretch. Muscle tissue is much like honey in that it becomes more pliable when it's warm, so the jogger (or tennis buff, aerobic dancer, etc.) who does his or her stretching before so much as lifting a finger risks tiny—and sometimes not so tiny—muscle tears. Hence, rule number one of safer stretching:

3

Always stretch a warm muscle, never a cold one.

That doesn't mean going through a full-scale workout before limbering up, but it does mean doing at least "a couple of minutes of light jogging to increase metabolic rate and core temperature," says William E. Prentice, Ph.D., coordinator of the Sports Medicine Program and assistant professor at the University of North Carolina. Not until such a warm-up has been completed should stretching of *any* type be attempted.

And what types of stretching are there?

There are three, basically: ballistic, static and PNF (propioceptive neuromuscular facilitation), which is a new type that is done with a partner and involves alternating contractions and stretching. But the best one for most people, these experts agree, is the static variety—a method that involves placing a given muscle in a "maximal position of stretch and holding it there for an extended period of time"—anywhere from 3 to 60 seconds, though about 30 seconds seems to be "as good a figure as any," Dr. Prentice says. Stretching of this type should be repeated three to four times for each muscle being stretched, he adds.

As for the ballistic stretching—the kind you may have learned in high school, where you lunge and bounce—all the experts agree that it's dangerous and should be shelved as the antique athletic maneuver that it is. Jerky movements can cause the very sort of muscle tears stretching is meant to prevent, which brings us to rule number two of safer stretching:

Stretch smoothly—never bounce.

Bouncing a stretch invites muscles to respond by tightening up to protect themselves, so the purpose of the stretch is defeated. Muscles prefer to be coaxed rather than jolted so, as you begin a stretch, do so slowly and smoothly, working toward a position that starts to feel tight but never becomes painful. Pain, in much the same way as bouncing, causes muscles to react by becoming *less* limber, not more. So use rule number three of safer stretching:

Pain in a stretch is self-defeating.

You're working *against* the body's loosening-up mechanisms by arousing pain during a stretch. Always ease yourself into a stretch, and hold it only as long as it feels comfortable. To do otherwise is to invite injury. And comfort leads us into rule number four of safer stretching:

Don't feel that preworkout stretching is absolutely necessary. If what you're stretching *for* is something short of a ballet routine or a feverish, 100-yard sprint, stretching might not even be necessary, these experts were willing to concede. As sportsmedicine practitioner and author Richard H. Dominguez, M.D., told the NSCA symposium, "I do not believe that stretching is necessary at all before jogging, but warm-up would be exceedingly important before any type of sprinting. The more explosive or powerful the activity, the more important the warm-up."

So unless you're exploding in your fitness efforts, don't get blown out of shape about feeling you have to stretch. If you wouldn't mind stretching *after* your workout, however, these experts agree that there are undeniable benefits to be gained from that. It seems stretching after a workout can clear exercise by-products (which can cause soreness if not cleared), and postworkout stretching can help prevent pooling of blood in exercised muscles as well. There is a tendency to be able to relax more *mentally* when stretching after a workout, too, the experts agree. It seems many of us tend to rush the stretching process when we've got our minds on the workout that looms ahead. It's certainly easier to relax — which is what stretching is all about — when the "hard" part is over. (For a more detailed warm-up and cool-down routine, see chapter 8.)

Start Your Day with a Stretch

Body and soul need a little time to cross the threshold from sleep to wakefulness. The easiest way to begin is simply to wiggle your fingers and toes while under the covers until you're ready for more serious undertakings. A more involved routine was developed by the Kripalu Center for Yoga and Health in Lenox, Massachusetts. The great thing about it is that you don't even have to get out of bed (though you may have to lie across it diagonally).

Here's how to start your day, the Kripalu way.

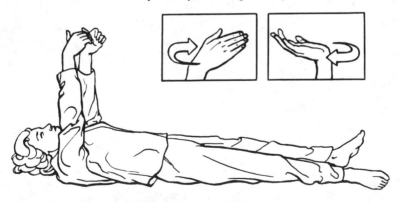

1. Remain in bed, or gently rise and lie on your back on the floor beside the bed. Slowly raise your arms vertically, rotate your wrists in both directions, then gently lower your arms.

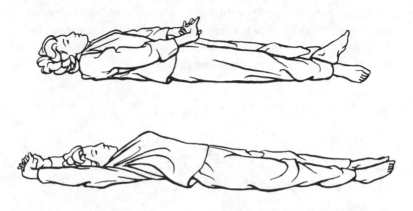

2. Clasp your hands on your stomach. Invert your palms so that they face your feet and stretch them downward. Now slowly (all of these movements should be done slowly) begin to lift your hands into the air, breathing in deeply and slowly and bringing them down to the floor behind or above your head, arms fully stretched out. Exhaling, stretch and arch your back, loosening your spine.

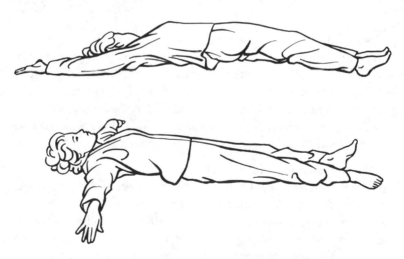

3. Unclasp your hands. Now, while inhaling, stretch your right arm and right leg in opposite directions so that they form a straight line, making the right side of your body longer than the left, while lifting your right hip. Relax and exhale. Now do the same with your left arm

and leg. Stretch them fully, inhaling deeply while lifting and twisting your left hip. Exhale, slowly bring your arms down, and extend them straight out from your body at shoulder height, touching the bed or floor. Relax for a moment, breathing deeply.

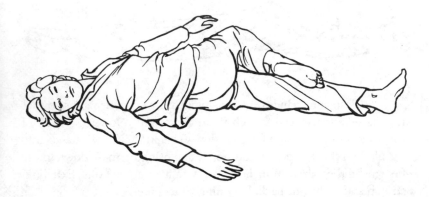

4. Inhaling, slowly raise your right knee, sliding your right foot along until it is next to your left knee. Exhaling slowly, twist your body, bringing your right knee over toward the bed or floor outside of your left thigh. As you do that, turn your head slowly to the right. Don't strain. Be very relaxed and enjoy the stretch. Now, exhaling, slowly go back to the center and slide your foot back to its starting position beside the other foot. Relax, then repeat with the other side.

5. This exercise, which is very good for people who suffer from tight back muscles, must be done on the floor, preferably on a thick, soft carpet. First, gently come to a sitting position with your knees up to your chest and your feet on the floor. Your hands are clasped around your knees, and your head is bent forward. Now begin to rock back onto your shoulders, keeping your spine well curved and your head tucked in so that your whole body is rolled up in a kind of ball. Rock backward and forward like this perhaps a dozen times fairly briskly, so that the momentum helps keep you going. Breathe in as you rock back and out as you rock forward. Then relax on your back.

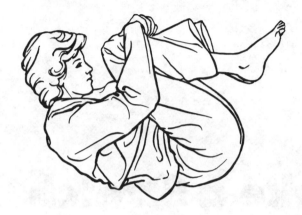

If you don't have time to do the five exercises we've described here, there is one quick way of easing out of bed in the morning. Simply bring your knees up to your chest, lock your arms around your shins, hold for a few seconds, and then lower your legs. Repeat several times. (This is an abbreviated version of the last stretch.)

Remember, during the time you are asleep, your body is in a kind of minihibernation. Your temperature actually goes down, and your circulation and breathing become sluggish. So take time to limber up before getting up, particularly if you wake up stiff.

Take a Stretch Break instead of a Coffee Break

If Phil Dunphy had his way, people would regularly break the sedentary workplace habits to which their bodies have grown accustomed. But that doesn't mean just practicing a regular fitness program. Even three or four good hours of exercise a week—a goal many of us strive for—aren't going to fully reverse the ravages of 40 to 50 hours of sitting behind a desk, believes the physical therapist, who runs the Institute of Health, Exercise and Athletic Rehabilitation in Red Bank, New Jersey.

To fight the inevitable aches and pains those who have desk jobs suffer, Dunphy believes you've got to regularly break a few physical habits on the job, in addition to getting your away-from-the-office exercise. "Many people don't understand the power of their jobs—how they can control their physical lives," says Dunphy.

But Dunphy isn't asking people to race around their offices all day. All he advocates is that periodically, throughout each and every day, you perform simple stretching exercises that reverse the muscle positions you're usually locked into on the job. Muscle aches and pains are often caused because you let muscles get into a rut—or habit—that after a prolonged time begins to hurt.

Nowhere are those aches more apparent for most desk-bound people than in the back, neck and shoulders. So here are Phil Dunphy's suggestions for quick and simple ways to break body habits in those areas.

Help for Your Aching Back

Most of the common backaches experienced by people who sit all day result from slumping over the desk with the back rounded, says Dunphy. So he believes that people need to perform stretches that gently *arch* the back—to reverse that bad habit. (Rounded-back stretches, like the one where you lie on the floor and bring your knees to your chest, are also beneficial, says Dunphy. But they're not enough.)

Here are three stretches that will gently arch your back. You'll probably want to do the second and third ones with your office door closed. If that's not possible, you might save them to do in the morning and evening.

Standing Arch.   Standing anywhere, place your hands on your buttocks and gently arch your back. Variation: Lean your back against a wall, press your shoulders against it and arch your back.

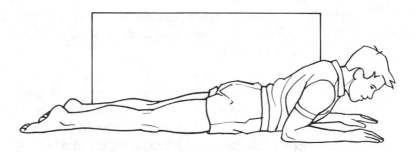

Modified Cobra.   Lying flat on your stomach, place your hands under your shoulders, then push up to an on-elbows position while keeping your hips on the floor.

A more advanced version of the Cobra is to push up onto your hands, straightening your arms while still keeping your hips on the floor.

The All-Fours Arch.   This is really the second half of what you might know as the "Angry Cat." On all fours, stretch upward into a rounded-back position, then sag downward into an arched-back position.

You can further promote good back posture by getting a chair that forces your back into a slight arch. Or you could use a lower-back cushion to do the same thing. Using back cushions or supports would also be a good idea when performing exercises on sit-down weight machines, says Dunphy.

Relief for Neck Pain

Most people aren't even aware of their neck—until it starts to hurt. Yet we can put an incredible strain on our neck, just hanging our head in what for us seems like a normal position, says Dunphy. What's the so-called normal position? You can check right now—are your ears and head hanging way out in front of your shoulders and body? That position can strain your neck. You should keep your head more centered over your body.

Also, just by the nature of office work, you're probably not accustomed to stretching your neck muscles anywhere *but* forward. So here are some quick exercises you can do anytime to develop a repertoire of movements to save you from neck ache.

Turtle Stretch.   Center your head in a straight position over your body, then pull your head back toward your shoulders. You should feel a pulling sensation in your neck.

Neck Rotation.   Place your left hand on your right shoulder and apply downward pressure. Turn your chin toward your left shoulder and continue to maintain pressure on your right shoulder until you feel a pull in the side of your neck. Then reverse the exercise.

Push and Pull.   This is a variation of the previous exercise. Grip your right arm (near the crook) with your left hand and pull your arm down gently. While pulling, bring your left ear toward your left shoulder, but do not turn your head.

No More Stiff Shoulders

Let's not forget the third important set of muscles that our daily sitting habits can wreak havoc on—the shoulders. "Executives work in close motion all the time," says Dunphy, "so their shoulders are almost always forward and down. Is it any wonder then that when they try to do an extreme motion, such as bringing their arm back to hit a tennis ball, they wind up hurting themselves?"

Dunphy thinks the shoulders should come in for their share of reverse stretching, too. The following exercises will not only relieve tension at work but also help prepare you for your tennis or racquetball game.

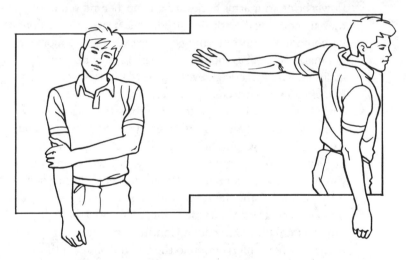

Back Shoulder Stretch.   Hold your right elbow with your left hand. Straighten your forearm out in front of you. With your left hand still holding your elbow, stretch your arm out in front of you and then across your body to the left. Repeat on the other side.

Front Shoulder Stretch.   Stand beside a wall with your arm straight out behind you. The underside of your arm should be flush against the wall. Slowly turn your body until it is perpendicular to the wall. Keep your arm (up to your shoulder) against the wall, and stretch as far as is comfortable. Repeat on the other side.

Hands Touching. Reach behind your head with one hand and behind your back with the other hand. Try to have your hands meet, but go only as far as is comfortable for you. Reverse your hands' positions and repeat.

"Little things, like doing these stretches throughout the day, do count," says Dunphy. "You're using your muscles differently than you normally do—and that's got to keep you more comfortable."

Here are a few other tips to stretch your tight, tense, corporate musculature.

- Stand erect with your arms behind your back, hands lightly clasped together. Slowly bend forward. At the same time slowly bring your arms backward and up behind you until they are pointing directly overhead, or as near as can be done without force. This refreshing exercise takes only a moment but makes you feel as though you've had a long rest. In addition, when practiced several times daily, it is a great help in maintaining more erect posture.

- The Circle is another exercise swing that stretches and stimulates your whole body. It's a great wake-up exercise and a wonderful invigorator during the day. Stand upright and bring your lightly clasped hands over your head, centering your head between your arms. Breathing deeply, bend your body sideways to the right, keeping your head centered between your arms. Continue to move slowly to the right, then forward toward the floor. Continue in a sweeping motion without interruption to the left and on up until you are in an upright position. Repeat in the opposite direction.

- Get into the habit of pacing. Instead of dropping into a chair to mull over a problem, get up and move around. As a general rule, never sit for more than an hour and a half without standing, stretching, and walking or pacing for at least five minutes. You'll go back to what you were doing refreshed, and you'll be more efficient.

- One of our favorite upright "stretchers" is walking in place through a doorway with your arms stretched overhead and your fingers touching the top of the door frame. This is marvelously stimulating, for it pulls everything from the ankles right up to the rib cage and shoulders. Even the neck receives a beneficial massage, for you can feel the pull and surge. Try it and feel the exhilaration. It is also an excellent way to help overcome tension.

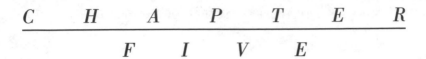

C H A P T E R
F I V E

Defuse Auto Tension

Okay, you've made it to work safely and calmly, but you still feel lethargic and kinked up from your ride. There are two great ways to "de-car." You can either take a brisk five-minute walk, which will get more oxygen into your system and make your muscles looser, or you can do a few simple exercises in your office.

Stretches to Uncramp and "De-Car" Your Body

These exercises are recommended by Charles T. Kuntzleman, Ed.D., national program director of Fitness Finders, Spring Arbor, Michigan. They are from his book *Maximum Personal Energy.*

Calf Tendon Stretcher. Stand two to three feet from a wall. Lean forward, keeping your body straight. Place your palms against the wall at eye level, then step backward. Continue to support your weight with your hands. Remain flat-footed until you feel your calf muscles stretching.

16

Side-to-Side Stretch.   Stand with your feet shoulder-width apart, with your left hand at your side and your right hand extended over your head. Slowly bend at the waist toward your left, reaching down your leg with your left hand. Try to get your upper body parallel to the floor. Hold for eight to ten seconds, then repeat in the other direction.

Simple Neck Stretches.   Stand or sit with your back straight, facing directly ahead. Slowly tilt your head up as if to look at something on the ceiling. After holding that position for ten seconds, turn and look over your left shoulder without twisting your upper body. Hold for ten seconds, then turn to the right. Again, hold, then look down, trying to touch your chin to your chest. This exercise can be practiced several times throughout the day and is a great way to reduce neck muscle tension that can lead to headaches.

Shoulder Stretch.   Grasping your elbows, lift your arms over your head. Drop your left hand down to your shoulder blade. Still grasping your left elbow, slowly pull it behind your head. Do not force. Hold, then repeat the motions on the other side.

Bend and Stretch.   While standing, clasp your hands behind your waist. As you slowly bend forward at the waist, lift your arms, keeping your elbows straight. When you begin to feel slight pressure in your arms and back, stop and hold. Return to the starting position.

And have a good day!

Don't Let Air Travel Crimp Your Style

When was the last time you arrived at your hotel from the airport feeling refreshed, relaxed and ready to start your business appointments? What, you laugh, is that a joke? Air travel seems destined to make aching, grouchy bears of us all. Between the mad dash through the airport, the inevitable delays and the heavy luggage, we're tired before we get on the plane. Then, just to add insult to injury, there's the typical airplane seat, a form of torture just short of The Rack.

It's no wonder so many people head for the bar upon arrival. But fitness experts say it doesn't have to be that way. While they can't promise your flight will be on time or your car won't break down on the way to the airport, they do have some suggestions to help you protect and limber up those achy, unused muscles.

Stretches for Jet-Setters

Gilda Marx, a West Coast fitness expert who franchises exercise salons throughout the United States, has developed a set of jet maneuvers, which she has already demonstrated to passengers in the air. Many of her maneuvers are designed to keep you as unobtrusive as possible, so you don't have to worry about curious stares from your fellow travelers.

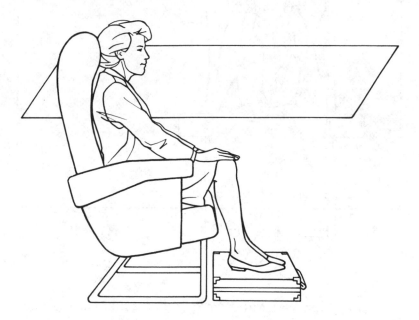

Sitting.   Keep your knees higher than your hips. This will relieve pressure and strain on your back. If there's no rung in front of you, use your briefcase to put your feet up. Avoid sitting on a bulky wallet. It can press on the sciatic nerve and give you leg pains. Finally, get up and walk around as much as you can.

Shoulder Tension Reliever.   Rotate your shoulders forward, then backward. Then lift them up to your ears.

Foot Flexer.   Take your shoes off and wiggle your toes. Rotate your ankles clockwise, then counterclockwise.

Leg Stretcher.   With your toes on the floor, raise your heels.

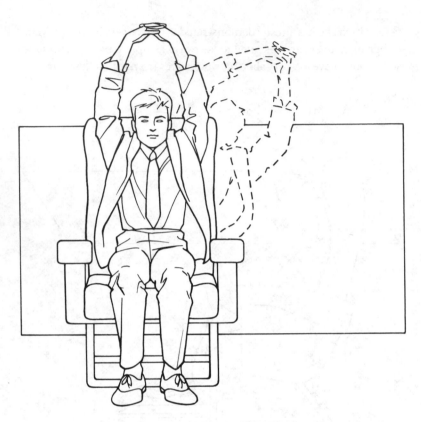

Shoulder, Waist and Arm Stretchers. Lift your hands over your head and lean to each side. A more complicated stretch: Put your arms above your head and grasp your elbows with opposite hands. Bring your chin in toward your neck, keeping your body centered and your hips down. Gently stretch to the right for three counts, then to the left.

Arm Strengthener. Put both hands on the seat in front of you with your arms outstretched, then push. Hold for five seconds and release.

Inner Thigh Strengthener. Make a fist, place your hand between your knees and squeeze.

Abdomen Strengthener. Inhale and pull your stomach muscle toward the back. Hold for four seconds, then exhale.

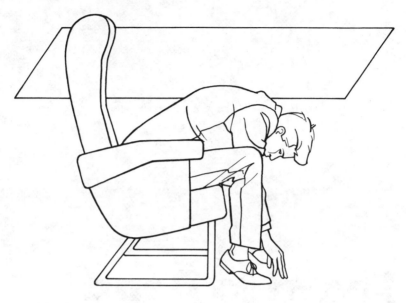

Back Stretcher. This one can be done under the guise of looking for something in your briefcase. Bring your head down and your knees up until they meet. Hold for five seconds and relax.

Learn to Bend

Ooo-aaahhhh!

This is the distressing cry of a common species seen throughout the world: the bending-twisting-reaching person who is bending-twisting-reaching the wrong way. The baleful shriek usually signals the onset of pain, the start of disability and the realization that some stupid act has just been committed.

Smarter — and Safer — Ways to Reach and Bend

At one time or another we've all hurt our muscles, bones and backs for the sake of the long reach or the big bend. Is such grief the inevitable fate of the body human?

Probably. But medical experts contend that it's possible to prevent many, if not most, of these injuries by teaching your body a thing or two about proper movement. Some authorities are quick to point out that there's a right way and a wrong way to drag a spare tire out of a car trunk, climb out of a lounge chair, stuff a briefcase into an airplane's overhead compartment or perform any other muscle-defying feat.

22

So we present some of their recommendations on sensible movement—a guide to bending, twisting and reaching in everyday life. But remember: These suggestions, though particularly useful for people with back and muscle problems, are no substitute for proper exercise and professional care.

The experts we consulted included Augustus A. White III, M.D., professor of orthopedic surgery at Harvard Medical School; Carl Granger, M.D., head of the department of rehabilitation medicine at Buffalo General Hospital in Buffalo, New York; Lydia Wingate, Ph.D., coordinator of the rehabilitation department at Buffalo General; Michael Wolf, Ph.D., a New York City fitness consultant; William Grana, M.D., director of the Oklahoma Center for Athletes at Presbyterian Hospital in Oklahoma City; and Dennis Zacharkow, physical therapist in the department of physical medicine and rehabilitation at the Mayo Clinic in Rochester, Minnesota.

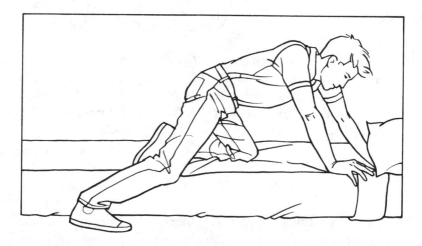

The Bedspread Crawl.   When you make the bed, you bend at the hips and reach out over it to smooth the covers—but this maneuver puts a lot of pressure on your spine. It's better to work kneeling on the bed with one knee, bracing yourself against the bed with one hand.

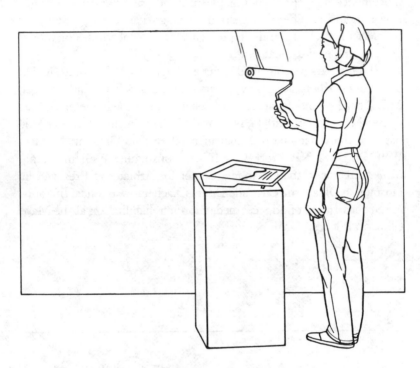

The Painter Principle.   To paint a room, stay as close as possible to what you're painting (don't overstretch because it seems easier than moving the ladder). Try to move your arms no lower than your waist and no higher than your shoulders, and use equipment (like rollers and paint guns) that let you avoid a lot of reaching.

The No-Backache Bow.   To empty the dishwasher, thumb through a low filing cabinet, check a roast in the oven, look for something on a bottom shelf or do anything else that requires a low profile, don't stand and bend at the waist. Simply lower yourself on one knee or squat down, as shown at top on the opposite page.

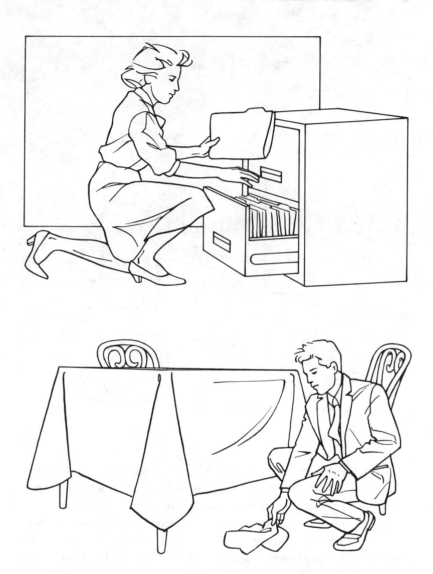

The Dinner-Hour Dip.   You drop your napkin in a restaurant. How do you retrieve it without banging your chin on the table, pulling a muscle or making your dinner partner wish you were at the next table? You should not do what comes naturally—bend over and reach while sitting. Instead, get out of your chair and squat down to reach the napkin, keeping your spine rigid and as upright as possible.

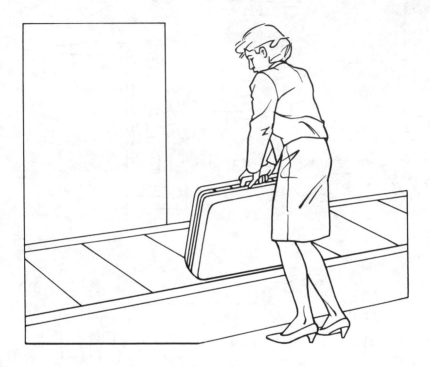

The Airport Lift. You're in the baggage-claim area of the airport, and your suitcase is circling on the luggage carousel. How are you going to get your suitcase without straining your back or knocking a fellow traveler to the floor? Stand as close to the suitcase as possible, bend at the hips and the knees, tense up your lower back muscles and slowly pull the bag toward you. Don't jerk it and don't lift it vertically.

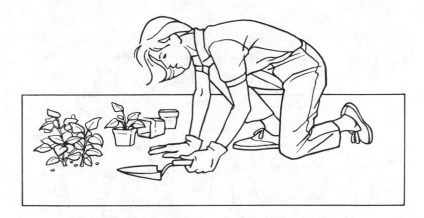

The Gardening Maneuver. Bow to the limitations of the human body: Rather than enduring a back-breaking stoop in the standing position, do your gardening on one or both knees, supporting your weight, if necessary, with one hand on the ground. Use short-handled tools if you want, and use cushioned knee pads.

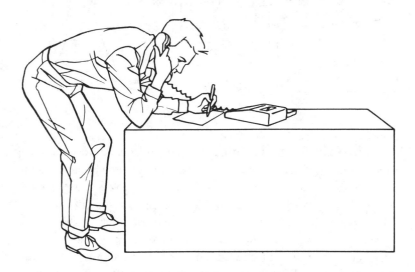

The Tabletop Prop. If you must bend over while standing to write on a desk or tabletop, do two things: (1) Bend at your knees as well as at your hips; and (2) prop yourself on the writing surface with your hand or elbow.

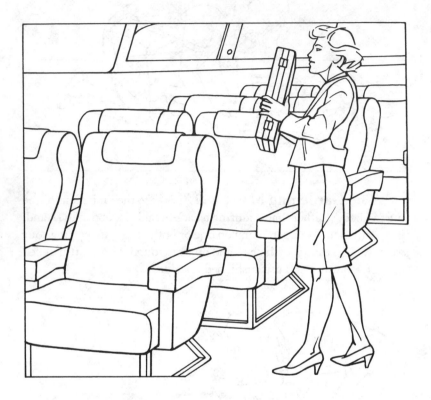

The Overhead Juggle.   On an airplane, how do you heave your carry-on luggage into those overhead compartments without straining every muscle in your body? For one thing, don't try to *heave* anything — lift slowly and steadily instead. And if possible, avoid lifting heavy objects over your head. Otherwise, tense your back, stand just beneath the compartment, hold the load close to your body and lift it in increments — first to your chest, then above your shoulders, then into the compartment. Reverse the procedure to get your luggage down.

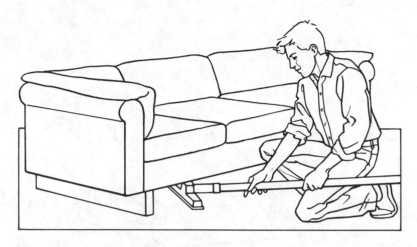

The Vacuum-Cleaner Curtsy.   Don't try to vacuum under couches and other pieces of furniture from a hunched position. Instead, get down on one knee and use a long-handled vacuum cleaner. If necessary, wear knee pads.

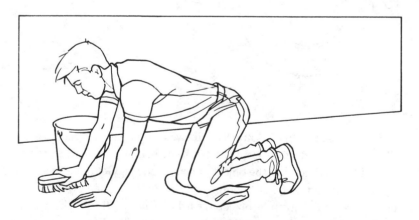

The Lowdown on Scrubbing.   If you don't do windows but occasionally scrub floors, try not to scrub them while sitting on your heels and bending forward. Instead, get down on all fours (with a towel under your knees to cushion them), keeping your head in line with your spine.

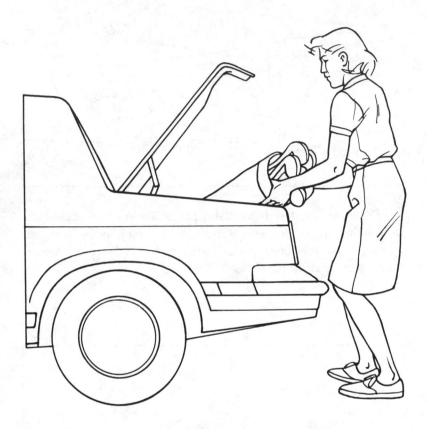

The Car-Trunk Caper.   To avoid ending up in traction, don't lift a heavy object out of your car trunk by bending forward from the lower back and holding the object at arm's length. Get as close as you can to the object, bend at the hips *and* the knees, tense up your lower back muscles and hoist the object toward you (not vertically), keeping it as close to your body as possible.

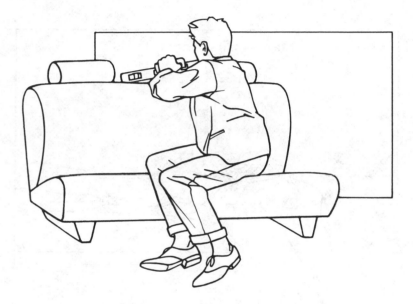

The Backseat Reach.   You're in the driver's seat of your car and your briefcase is in the backseat. Problem: How do you get the briefcase to the front seat without getting out of the car or twisting your body into an excruciating half nelson? Answer: While sitting, rotate your whole body 90 degrees to the right (or turn and rest your knees on the seat, facing the briefcase), then grasp the briefcase and pull it toward you—but don't try to lift it straight up.

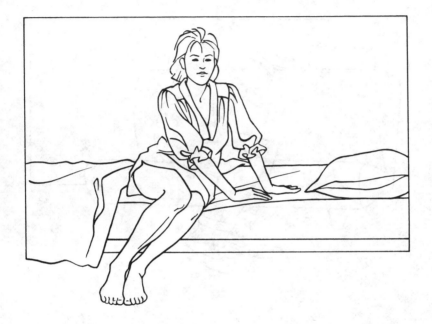

The Morning Swing.   In the morning, don't sit bolt upright and try to pop out of bed like a jack-in-the-box. That can be tough on your spine. Instead, roll over onto your side facing the edge of the bed and prop yourself up on your elbow. Swing your legs over the side of the bed and push yourself into a sitting position with your hands. Then use your hands to push against the bed as you get to your feet.

The Beach-Chair Shuffle.   To extract yourself from a lounge chair (or any low chair), first scoot forward to the chair's edge and tuck your heels back toward the front of the chair as far as they'll go, as shown at top on the opposite page. Then stand up, pushing off with your arms.

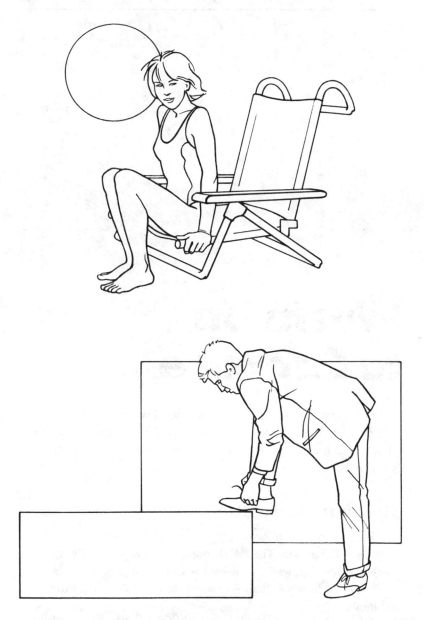

The Shoestring Trick.   If you have to tie your shoe, don't bend over while standing to reach your feet. You're asking for back trouble. Either get down on one knee or stand while resting your foot on a chair.

Warm Up to Exercise

Cold, stiff muscles and tendons are never ready to spring immediately into action, no matter how in shape you are. You must warm and stretch muscles and get your blood moving before you start *any* vigorous activity.

Start with Relaxation

Begin warming up by doing the simple relaxation technique shown in the first illustration. Then work into your activity gradually. If you're going to run or jog, walk slowly for five to ten minutes. If you're going to cycle, cycle slowly at first. A gradual start also stimulates the heart and lungs.

If your back and shoulder muscles feel tight, do stretches 2 and 3. If your arm and back muscles feel stiff, do stretches 4, 5, 6 and 9. If your leg or calf muscles feel tight, do stretches 7, 8, 10 and 11. Always stretch any muscle that's ever given you trouble in the past.

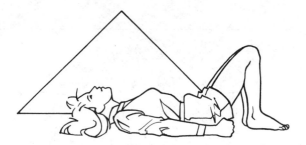

1. Relaxation.   Lie on the floor with your knees bent and arms outstretched. Take several long, slow, deep breaths. Clench your fists for two or three seconds and release.

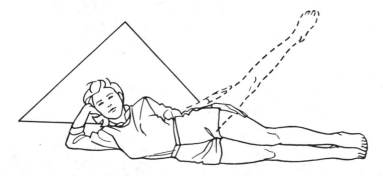

2. Lower Back and Hip Stretcher.   Lie on your back with your knees straight. Raise one knee to your chest. Grasp your leg just below the knee and pull the knee toward your chest. Hold for five seconds, then curl your head and shoulders toward the knee. Hold five seconds longer. Repeat with your other leg. Exercise each leg four times.

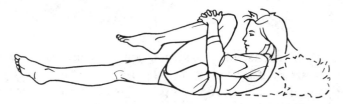

3. Side Leg Raises.   Lie on your side with your head resting on your hand and your feet together. Raise your upper leg from the floor, keeping it straight with the toes pointed. Lower your leg to the starting position. Alternate sides and repeat ten times with each leg.

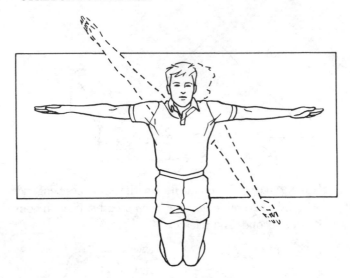

4. Windmills. Kneel, keeping your waist and back straight. With your arms outstretched to the sides, lean to one side. Place your lower hand as close to the floor as possible while raising your other hand. Return to the starting position and lean to the other side. Repeat eight times on each side.

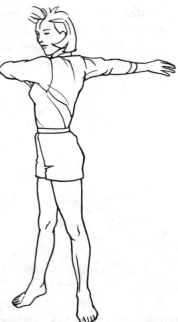

5. Trunk Twister. Stand with your feet shoulder-width apart, with your arms extended to the sides at shoulder level. Keeping your heels on the floor, slowly twist your torso to one side as far as you can. Return to the starting position, then twist slowly to the other side. Repeat for a total of six complete twists.

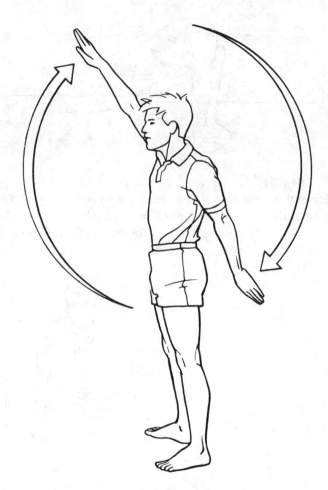

6. Arm Circles.   Stand with your feet shoulder-width apart.
Swing your arms forward, making large sweeping circles. Repeat ten
times, then reverse the swing and repeat ten more times.

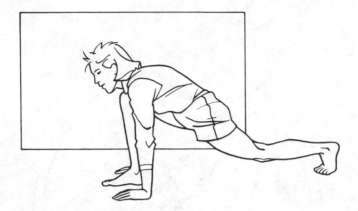

7. Forward Lunge.   With your palms on the floor, move one foot forward so that it is flexed under your chest and your knee is directly over the ankle. Stretch your other leg out behind you. Roll your body forward while pushing your hips toward the floor. *Don't bounce.* Hold for five seconds or longer. Reverse legs and repeat. Stretch each leg five times.

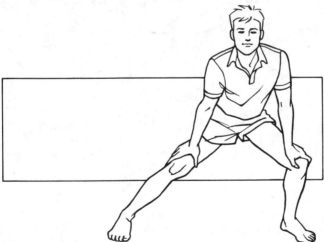

8. Side Lunge.   Spread your legs in a wide straddle position, with your toes pointing straight ahead. Shift your weight to one side so that most of your weight is on one leg. *Don't bounce.* Hold this position for five seconds or longer. Shift your weight to your other leg and repeat. Repeat four times on each side.

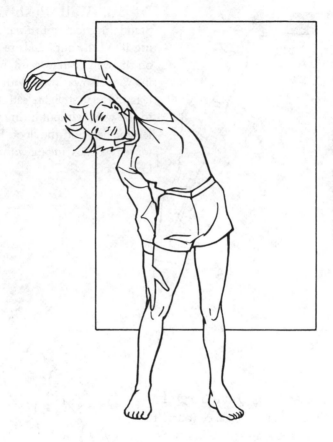

9. Side Stretch I.   Stand with your feet shoulder-width apart, with one arm extended upward (palm facing inward) and the other arm extended downward (palm touching the outside of your thigh). Lean to that side, sliding your hand down your leg as far as you can comfortably reach. Switch arms and repeat on the other side. Do this stretch six times on each side.

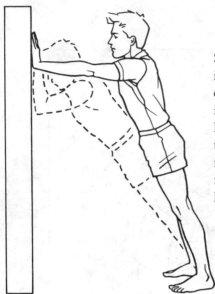

10. Wall Push-Ups.
Stand three feet from a wall, facing it. With your hands resting on the wall, lean forward, bending your elbows slowly. With your legs and torso straight, lean closer to the wall, without lifting your feet or heels off the floor. Hold for ten seconds. Repeat with your knees bent.

11. Standing Quad Stretcher.
Stand erect and balance yourself with your hand against a wall or chair. Bend one knee, grasp that ankle and draw the leg up and back. Hold. Pull your foot gently until you feel slight discomfort in your upper front thigh. Hold for five seconds or longer. Repeat with your other leg.

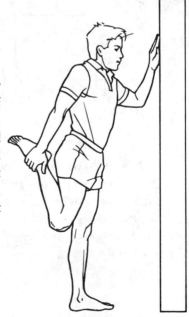

After Each Workout

When you're finished working out, don't stop abruptly and dash for the shower. Cooling your muscles is just as important as warming them up.

Keep moving for another five to ten minutes, tapering off gradually. Walking is the easiest way to cool down—it helps your muscles pump blood from your arms and legs back to the heart and brain and allows your heart rate and blood pressure to return to normal.

To complete the cool-down phase, do exercises 1 through 11, *in reverse order.* This will prevent your muscles from locking into a contraction or spasms, so they will be limber, not stiff, the next day. In fact, the more you stretch *after* each workout, the less you'll need to stretch before your next session.

More Stretches

To add variety to your stretching routine, substitute these ten stretches for the first group. Don't forget the relaxation step! And take a deep breath after each stretch.

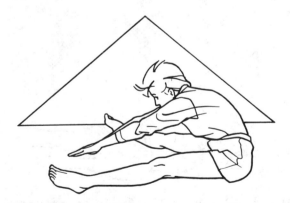

1. Sitting Stretch.   Sit on the floor with your legs extended at least six to ten inches apart. Bend forward with your arms outstretched as far as you can and hold the position for eight to ten seconds. Do not strain or bounce.

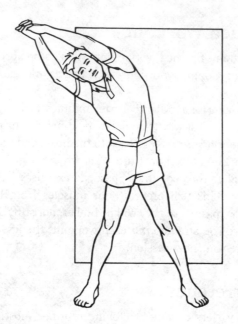

2. Side Stretch II.   Stand straight with your legs spread comfortably. Clasp your hands above your head. Lean from the waist to the right as far as is comfortable without moving your hip. Repeat, leaning to the left.

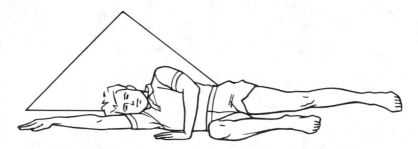

3. Pedal Stretch.   Lie on your right side with your head resting on your outstretched arm and the palm of your left hand on the floor in front of your chest. Raise your legs slightly off the floor and pedal for ten seconds as if you were riding a bicycle. Switch sides and repeat.

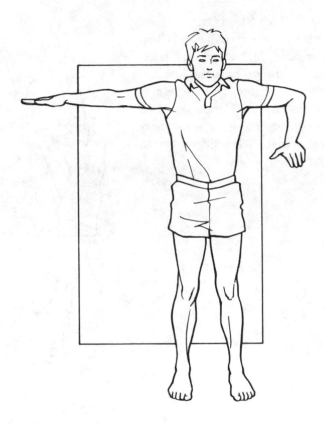

4. Arm Stretch.   Hold one arm straight out from your side, level with your shoulder. Make an arc by raising your arm straight up, then lowering it to your side. Hold your arm out again. Swing it across your chest as far as is comfortable. Swing it toward your back as far as it will comfortably go. Now hold your arm straight in front of you, bending your elbow at a right angle, with the palm toward the floor. Without moving your upper arm, move your forearm straight up and then straight down. Alternate arms.

5. Sky Stretch.   Stand with your feet spread apart. Clasp your hands high above your head. Lean your head back and look up. Stretch your shoulder muscles as if you were reaching for the sky. Hold for several seconds, or as long as is comfortable. Relax. Repeat two to four times.

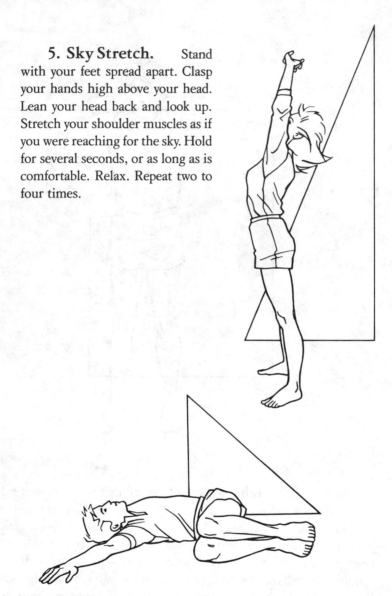

6. Knee Swing.   Lie on your back with your arms outstretched and your palms down. Keeping your ankles together, raise your knees to your chest and roll your knees to touch the floor, first on one side, then the other. Keep your hands and shoulders firmly on the floor. Repeat 15 to 30 times.

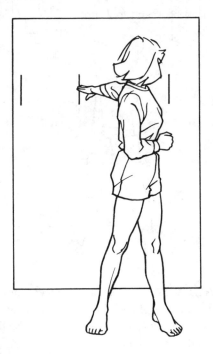

7. Side Twist.   Make three imaginary marks at shoulder height on a wall at about one-foot intervals. Stand with your back to the wall, an arm's length away. Extend one arm and twist your body, touching each mark with your hand. Reach as far as possible. Change sides and repeat.

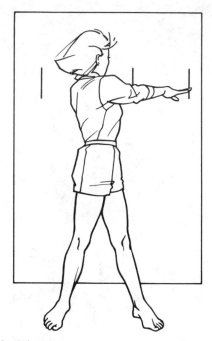

8. Double Twist.   Standing three feet from a wall, imagine three marks at shoulder height on the wall. With your back to the wall and your feet about two feet apart, bend and touch the floor. Straighten up. Twist your body and touch the marks. Return to the starting position and repeat, this time twisting to the other side.

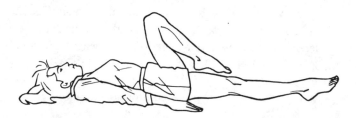

9. Horizontal Leg Stretch.   Lie on your back with both legs outstretched. Bend your right knee and raise it until your foot is a few inches off the floor. Keeping your hips straight, slide your left leg to the left along the floor. Slide it back and lower the other leg. Repeat, alternating legs.

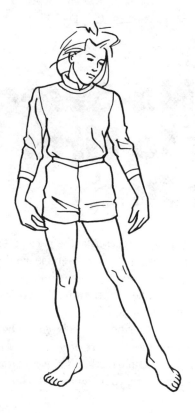

10. Leg Arc.   Stand straight with your arms at your sides. In one continuous motion, swing your leg straight out to one side. Swing it back across your other leg as far as comfortably possible. Return to the starting position and repeat with your other leg.

The No-Sweat Way to Firm Your Body

Ask a bunch of people to describe the perfect exercise and they'd probably all agree on a few points: The exercise would be easy; you'd be able to do it indoors when it's cold and wet outdoors; it wouldn't make you sweat; and it wouldn't take much time. Believe it or not, there *is* an exercise that fits that description: isometrics.

Isometrics involves tensing a muscle group by using it to exert steady pressure against another part of your body or an immovable object (like a wall). This simple method firms and tones your muscles, thus improving your posture, your figure and your strength.

When Push Comes to Shove

Isometrics was originally developed to help people who had injuries keep their muscle tone intact even though movement was painful or impaired. But you'll be able to use it to more easily tackle chores like opening stuck windows, shoveling snow and carrying packages. You'll also be able to firm those parts of you that have started to sag. Are your upper arms getting flabby? Tense them up once a day with the Doorway Press-Up. If a flatter tummy is your goal, smooth it with the Curl-Up. For firmer buttocks, simply tense them while you're reading or talking on the phone.

It may sound unlikely that you can benefit so much from doing something so simple. But thousands of people already have. In fact, Charles Atlas developed his he-man physique using a form of isometrics — and nothing else.

But although isometrics firms your muscles and builds strength, it doesn't improve endurance. Strength enables you to more easily lift, pull or push heavy loads for a *short* period of time; endurance enables you to be active for long periods of time. So keep up your endurance-building exercises like walking or jogging.

To do isometrics, you'll need a towel or a belt, a doorway and a chair. It's best to do them every day, either when you first get up, a half hour or so before you go to bed or during breaks at work.

When you first start your isometrics program, hold the following positions for only six seconds (count slowly to six). Then add one second each week until you reach ten. Apply steady pressure and don't start or finish with a sudden jerk. The most important thing to remember is to breathe throughout the exercise. Take a deep breath before tensing your muscles, then exhale slowly as you count. If you have trouble remembering to exhale, count out loud. That way you have no choice but to keep breathing. If you have heart problems or high blood pressure, you should check with your doctor before doing isometrics.

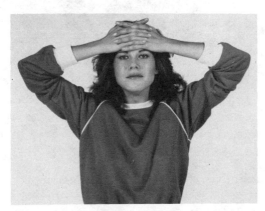

Brow Clasp.   Interlock your fingers and place your palms across your forehead. Press your head forward, resisting any movement by pressing backward with your hands. This strengthens and tones the neck muscles. This and the Head Clasp and Head Turn will help keep your neck looking young and firm.

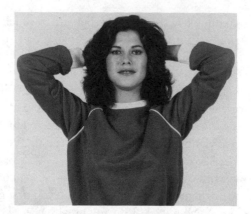

Head Clasp.   Place your interlocked hands at the base of your skull with your elbows held out wide. Press your head back and at the same time resist any movement by pressing your hands forward.

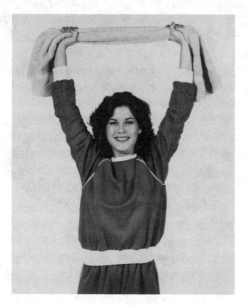

Overhead Pull-Out.   Grasp a belt or rolled-up towel so that when you pull tightly, your hands will be at the same width as your shoulders. In a standing position, raise your arms over your head and pull. This exercise works on your posture by strengthening your shoulders, chest, upper back and arms.

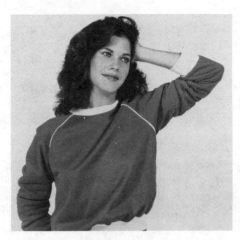

Head Turn.   Place the palm of your right hand at your right temple with your fingers pointing to the back of your head. Try to turn your head toward your hand while applying pressure from your hand and arm. Now do this on the left side.

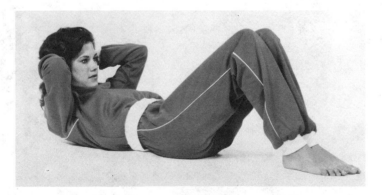

Curl-Up.   Lying on your back, place your heels on the floor by your buttocks. Lock your fingers behind your head and curl up by raising your head, shoulders and upper back off the floor. Hold this position for six seconds. This firms the abdominal muscles.

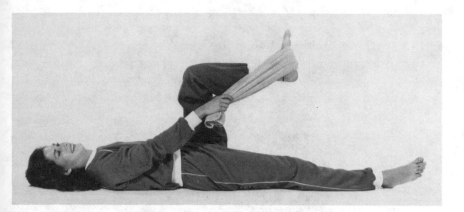

Leg Press.   Take either a belt or a rolled-up towel and loop it around the sole of your foot. Bring your knee up so that your upper leg is vertical to the floor. Pull the towel taut with your leg while pulling back with your arms. This is good for the hip and front of the upper leg. Repeat with your other leg.

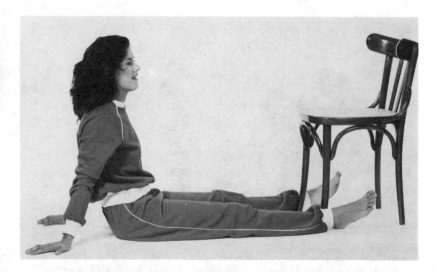

Leg Squeeze.   While sitting on the floor, grip the legs of a chair with your feet and squeeze hard inward as if you're trying to crush the chair. This works the inner thighs.

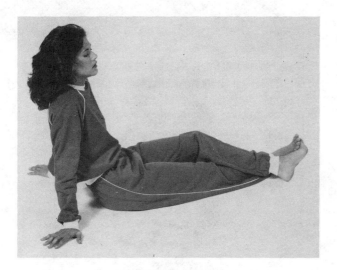

Leg Pull.   This is the reverse of the leg squeeze. Still sitting on the floor, cross your feet at your ankles and bring your legs firmly together. Try to pull your legs apart. But resist, of course. This smooths and firms the outer thighs.

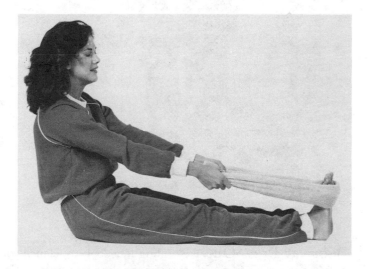

Feet Pointing.   Sitting with your legs straight out and the towel around the balls of your feet, try to push your toes away from you, but pull back hard on the towel. This exercise firms up your calves.

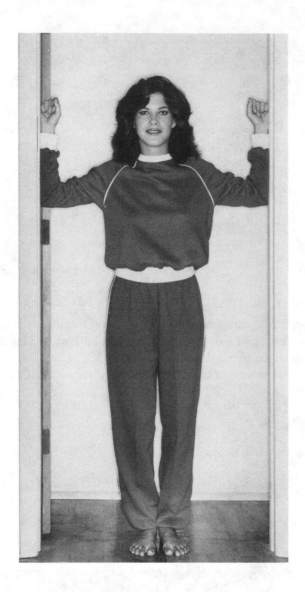

Doorway Press-Out. Standing in a doorway, clench your fists and press them against both sides of the door frame about level with the top of your head. This firms up the muscles at the back of your upper arms, as well as the upper back and chest.

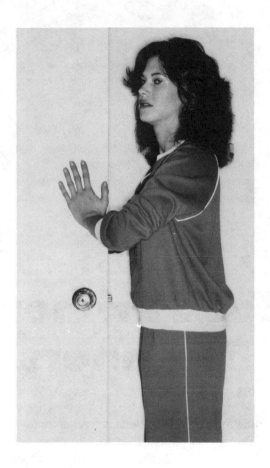

Doorway Press-In.   With your chest about four inches from the edge of an open door, bend your arms and push on both sides of the door with your palms toward each other. Then do this above your head by pushing your palms together. Both of these exercises shape and tone the chest muscles.

A Yoga Primer
for Beginners

Yoga is no longer thought to be a sideshow trick or the subject matter of exotic movies. It's a serious mental and physical discipline that many conventionally trained doctors think may help in both sickness and health. Fine. But what, *exactly*, is it? Basically, yoga teaches that a healthy person is a harmoniously integrated unit of body, mind and spirit. Therefore, good health requires a simple, natural diet, exercise in fresh air, a serene and untroubled mind and the awareness that man's deepest and highest self is identical with the spirit of God. As a result, to many devotees yoga becomes a philosophy that offers instruction and insight into every aspect of life: the spiritual, the mental *and* the physical. Of course, because it *is* all-encompassing, people who want to pick and choose from its smorgasbord can do so without being disappointed. Yoga is equally satisfying as a physical therapy alone.

An Ancient Method of Relaxing Away Tension

Yoga therapy begins with relaxation. Living in an age of anxiety, we are often unconscious of our tensions. With normal bodies, why are we depressed, tired, prey to disease? Because tension is invisibly draining away our health energies!

Ruth Rogers, M.D., of Daytona Beach, Florida, who has made a ten-year study of yoga therapy, says, "In understanding the healing process, relaxation is of supreme importance. You feel pain, and you don't want to move, so you tighten up. You're tense. Your muscles contract, constricting the blood flow. Swelling begins. More circulation is cut off, creating a vicious cycle. There's more pain, more tightening, more stiffness, more swelling . . . . This is also what happens in many back problems. But," she adds, "if you can relax, fresh blood can circulate nourishment to the afflicted tissues and relieve pain-loaded nerve endings. Healing can begin."

Most yoga therapy—some experts would claim *all* successful treatment—involves a three-pronged attack. When you practice yoga postures, you are strengthening the body. When you control your breathing, you are creating a chemical and emotional balance. And when you concentrate your mind on affirmations, you are practicing the power of prayer. But when all three approaches are synthesized, you are entering the most powerful mystery of healing: the basic harmony of life.

A Posture Program for Beginners

Before eating, in either the morning or the late afternoon, spread a blanket on the floor in a well-ventilated room. Wear loose clothing. As a general rule, backward-bending postures should be balanced by forward-bending poses.

Never force or strain in yoga. The postures should be performed slowly, even meditatively. Yoga postures are meant to be held in dynamic tension, and they should not be confused with vigorous calisthenics.

Twelve minutes of yoga a day will help produce a toning of the muscles and improved digestive, circulatory and respiratory systems. The following exercises will provide a well-balanced program, which

should be supplemented, of course, by any other postures that are
particularly good for your needs.

- First day: Complete Breath, Knee to Chest, Cobra, Corpse Pose.
- Second day: Complete Breath, Corpse Pose.
- Third day: Complete Breath, Bow, Cobra, Posterior Stretch,
  Corpse Pose.
- Fourth day and on: Repeat the sequence: First Day, Second
  Day, Third Day, and so forth.

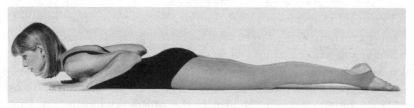

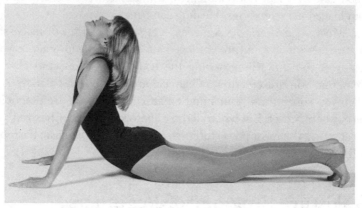

Cobra.   Lie on your stomach, toes extended. Place your hands,
palms down, under your shoulders on the floor. Inhaling, without
lifting your navel from the floor, raise your chest and head, arching
your back. Retain the breath, then exhale while slowly lowering to the
floor. Repeat one to six times.

Reported benefits: Tones the ovaries, uterus and liver. Aids in
relief and elimination of menstrual irregularities. Relieves constipation. Limbers the spine. Excellent for slipped disks.

Warning: Not recommended for sufferers of peptic ulcer, hernia
or hyperthyroid.

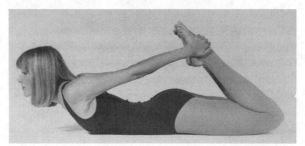

Bow. Lie flat on your stomach, grasping your ankles. Inhale. Lifting your legs, head and chest, arch your back into a bow. Retain the breath for a count of three, then exhale and lie flat. Repeat three or four times.

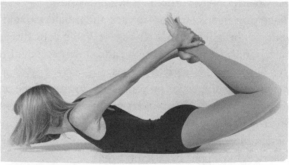

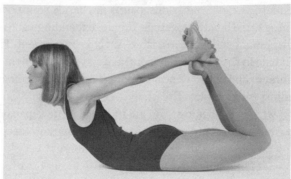

More advanced: While in the Bow position, rock back and forth, then from side to side. Slowly release and exhale.

Reported benefits: Massages the abdominal muscles and organs. Good for gastrointestinal disorders, constipation, upset stomach, sluggish liver. Reduces abdominal fat.

Warning: Not for persons suffering from peptic ulcer, hernia, or thyroid or endocrine gland disorders. Consult your doctor.

Complete Breath. Crowded city living, air pollution and sedentary jobs are helping to increase respiratory ailments. Tight clothes encourage shallow breathing and cramp the lungs. The purpose of the Complete Breath is to fully expand the air sacs of the lungs, thereby exposing the capillaries to the maximum exchange of carbon dioxide and oxygen.

1. Lie down and loosen your clothing. Place your hands on your abdomen and rest your fingertips lightly on your navel. Breathing through your nose, inhale and expand only your abdomen. (Your fingertips will meet.) Practice this Abdominal Breath slowly, without strain, ten times.
2. Place your hands on your rib cage and inhale, expanding only your diaphragm and your rib cage. (Watch your fingertips part.) Contract your diaphragm and slowly exhale. Practice this Diaphragm Breath ten times.
3. Placing your fingertips on your collarbones, inhale only in your upper chest. Your fingers will rise, indicating a shallow breath. This is how we usually breathe. Notice the insufficiency. Now raise your shoulders for more air. Exhale and practice this Upper Breath ten times.
4. Finally, placing your hands, palms up, beside your body, put these three breaths together. Inhale, expanding your abdomen, diaphragm and chest in a slow, wavelike movement. Hold. Exhale in the same order, contracting your abdomen, diaphragm and chest. Repeat these instructions to yourself as you adjust the Complete Breath to your own rhythm. Concentrate on what is happening: You are increasing the expansion of the terminal air sacs in your lungs. Notice how slow, deep breathing makes you calm, yet fills you with energy! Very logically, yoga traditionally links a long life with proper breathing.

Reported benefits: Increases vitality. Soothes the nerves. Strengthens flabby intestinal and abdominal muscles.

Corpse Pose. Lie down on your back in a quiet place. Place your arms beside your body, palms upturned. Keep your heels slightly apart. Breathe slowly and deeply, feeling a sense of relaxation come over your whole body. Concentrate on loosening all tensions.

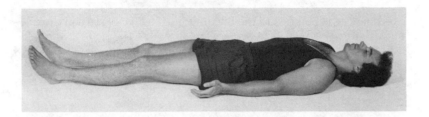

The following variation will increase your ability to relax:

1. While in the Corpse Pose, slowly inhale through your nostrils (always breathe through your nostrils during yoga, since the tiny hairs strain out impurities) and tense your ankles, feet and toes. Hold the breath while you tighten the muscles. Exhale and relax.
2. Slowly inhale and contract your kneecaps, calves, ankles, feet and toes. Hold and tighten. Exhale and relax.
3. Slowly inhale, contracting all the muscles of your abdomen, pelvic area, hips, thighs, kneecaps, calves, ankles, feet and toes. Hold the breath and tighten the muscles. Exhale and relax.
4. Inhale. Tense your neck, shoulders, arms and elbows, wrists, hands and fingers, chest muscles, and all the muscles down to your toes. Hold and tense. Exhale and relax.
5. Inhale and contract your scalp, the tiny muscles of your face and your forehead; tighten your tongue, constrict your throat and tighten your whole body. Hold and feel the tension. Exhale and relax. Now, let the strain melt into the floor. Feel heavy. Enjoy the support of the floor. Sense the tingling of fresh circulation, the new muscle tone and emotional calm.

Reported benefits: Stimulates blood circulation and exercises the inner organs. Alleviates fatigue, nervousness, neurasthenia (a general worn-out feeling), asthma, constipation, indigestion, insomnia, lumbago. Teaches mental concentration.

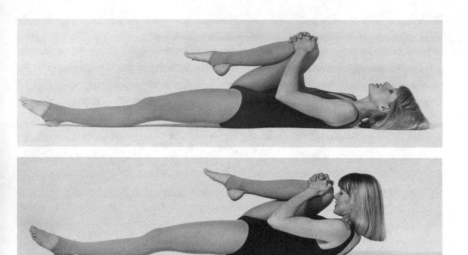

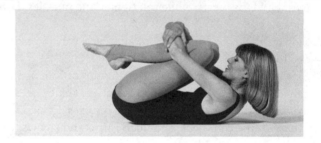

Knee to Chest.   Lying on your back, bring your knees to your chest. Grasping your folded knees, rock gently back and forth. (This relaxes and massages the spine.) Lower your legs one at a time. Inhale and bend your right knee to your chest, pulling it to your chest with interlocked fingers. Retain the breath and raise your head, touching your knee with your nose. Hold for a count of ten. Exhale and lower your head almost to the floor. Straighten your right leg and lower it slowly to the floor. Repeat five times, then change legs. Exhale as you lower your head to the floor. Repeat with your left leg. Now draw up both legs and touch your nose to your knees. Hold the breath. Exhale and relax.

Reported benefits: Relieves stiffness and soreness of the back and extremities. Relieves constipation, flatulence.

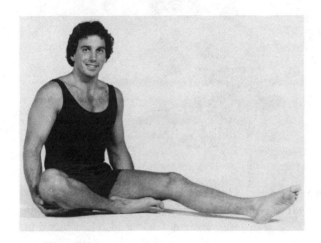

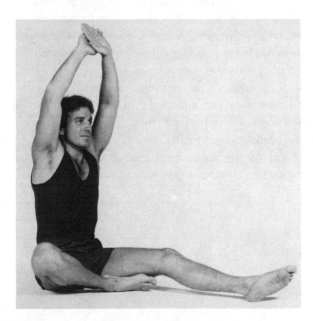

Posterior Stretch.   Sit on the floor with your left leg outstretched and your right heel tucked into your crotch. Inhale and reach

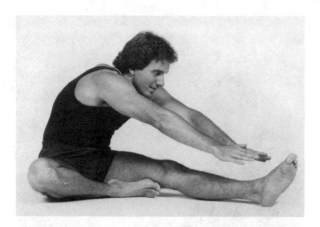

your arms overhead. Hold the breath and drop forward, reaching your arms toward your left ankle and lowering your head to your knee. (If you can only grasp your calf, do that and relax, breathing slowly.) Concentrate on the muscles as they slowly lengthen, and inch down lower. Close your eyes. Release any discomfort in a sensation of relaxation. Hold for one minute. Inhale, raise up with your arms overhead and exhale as you lower your arms to the side. Repeat with the opposite leg. Repeat with both legs outstretched.

Reported benefits: A powerful massage to the abdominal organs. Improves digestion and elimination through the forward-bending movement. Relaxes tensions in the back. Brings fresh circulation to the face, firming the tissue and improving color.

Warning: Not for those with slipped disks. It is important that the back is not rounded. All forward bends should be done from the hips.

C H A P T E R
E L E V E N

T'ai Chi Chu'an, the Natural Tranquilizer

T'ai Chi Chu'an, a unique system of exercise developed hundreds of years ago in China by Taoist monks, has recently been attracting the attention of American medical personnel and physical educators. In hospital tests, this exotic exercise has favorably impressed cardiologists as a form of activity that has potential in the treatment of heart patients. According to the Chinese, who have a much longer experience than Americans with T'ai Chi, its practice for 20 minutes a day over a period of years can prolong youthful vigor and rejuvenate the body.

The 108 basic moves or forms of T'ai Chi use every part of the body. Hands, elbows, fists, legs, shoulders, head, buttocks, feet, toes, sides of feet—even the eyes—are all brought into play in a pattern of continually flowing movement. The exercise is performed in a slow, almost leisurely manner, without any special muscular effort. And because it isn't strenuous, anyone from 8 to 80 can practice T'ai Chi safely.

A Calming Effect on Mind and Body

One test of T'ai Chi's effect on the heart was made at Montefiore Hospital in New York City. Lenore Zohman, M.D., chief of physical therapy, took an electrocardiogram of a well-known T'ai Chi teacher, Sophia Delza, the foremost woman instructor of T'ai Chi in the Western world. Although it is normally the case that exercise increases the heart rate, the cardiogram on Delza indicated that her heart rate was not changed when she practiced T'ai Chi. While laypeople might not be impressed, doctors appreciate the rare value of an activity that does not put stress on the heart, and they are alert to its therapeutic possibilities. According to Louis Brinberg, M.D., formerly a cardiologist at New York's Mount Sinai Hospital, "It will be interesting to see what can be done with T'ai Chi when used as an adjunct to the usual therapy for cardiac patients."

The value of T'ai Chi seems to stem as much from its psychological as from its physiological effects. The fact that modern medicine is finding more and more connections between mental attitudes and physical health may indeed help to explain the value of T'ai Chi, which is designed to have a calming effect on the mind and nervous system.

A Natural Tranquilizer

It has been quite conclusively demonstrated that T'ai Chi has a tranquilizing effect on the emotions. The overburdened executive, the harassed housewife, the uptight student, the anxious clerk—all might discover that a ten-minute break for a round of T'ai Chi can put them in a better frame of mind and help them to bear the pressures of everyday living without ulcers or nervous breakdowns.

Probably the most difficult T'ai Chi principle for a beginner to follow is the one of complete relaxation. Most Westerners attack daily exercise as though they were wrestling with a bear. They don't really enjoy doing it.

By contrast, T'ai Chi requires that you relax your facial muscles, shoulders, abdomen and thighs, and follow the shifting pattern of movements with a light, calm mind. Eventually you will experience a sensation almost like floating.

By their very nature, all of the movements of T'ai Chi are geared to encourage relaxation. The weight of the body shifts continuously from one foot to the other, and the movements are performed in circles, arcs and spirals. The end of each movement becomes the beginning of the next one, which conserves energy and produces a feeling of tranquility and emotional security.

In order to perform the exercises properly, the body must move as a unit. This principle of unity in movement is one of the ways in which T'ai Chi contrasts most basically to Western calisthenics, which use various parts of the body independently. Robert J. Rogers, Ph.D., a Chappaqua, New York, psychologist, psychoanalyst and T'ai Chi practitioner, believes that T'ai Chi, "practiced correctly over a long period of time, creates a kind of protective psychological shield that helps a person combat stress, which is one of the main causes of disease."

The Inner Strength of *Chi*

At the heart of T'ai Chi is the Chinese concept of *chi,* a word of many meanings—air, vitality, spirit, breath, atmosphere and circulation. It is hard to define *chi.* One T'ai Chi expert calls it "biophysical energy generated by respiratory rhythm." Perhaps the best English equivalent is "intrinsic energy," or "vital force." Whatever *chi* is, doctors of Chinese medicine say it can be cultivated through practice of the exercise and stored in a spot called the *tan-t'ien,* located exactly three inches below the navel. Once stored, the *chi* can be circulated by the mind throughout the body. In an ancient Chinese treatise on T'ai Chi, the author states, "The mind directs the *chi,* which sinks deeply and permeates the bones. The *chi* circulates freely, mobilizing the body so that it heeds the direction of the mind. If the *chi* is correctly cultivated, your spirit of vitality will rise, and you will feel as though your head were suspended by a string from above."

Performing T'ai Chi

The T'ai Chi postures that follow are just a few of the many that may be practiced.

When you perform these exercises, remember that the body always moves as one unit. This rule applies to all T'ai Chi movements. And when you move as one unit, you should notice that your body's awkwardness will be greatly reduced. In its place, you should experience a gracefulness that aids in your inner circulation of *chi*.

This gracefulness can be thought of as the outer expression of *chi*. You probably can't really experience the inner peace connected with *chi* without this outward grace. The external relaxation you radiate is a reflection of the inner peace you are creating. Awkward movements, on the other hand, will only disrupt the *chi*'s flow.

Move slowly, without any visible effort.

Beginning of T'ai Chi

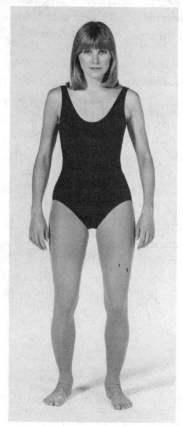
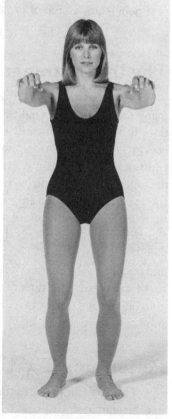

1. Stand relaxed, with your elbows and knees *slightly* bent.

2. Raise your arms *slowly* to shoulder height.

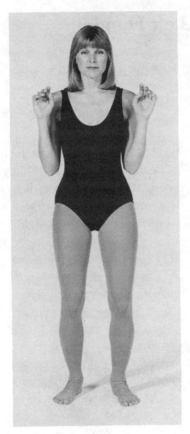

3. Draw back your arms by bending your elbows.

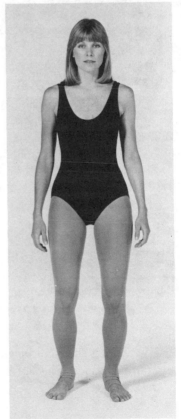

4. Let your arms sink *gently* to your sides. You are again in the beginning position.

Note: Do not exert force, but let your arms rise as though they were floating up from underwater to the surface. In the same way, let them fall to your sides again without strain. Concentrate on total relaxation.

Ward Off with Your Left Hand

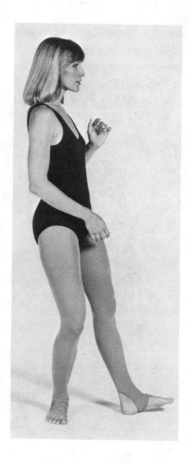

1. This movement follows "Beginning of T'ai Chi." Shift your weight to your left foot, then turn on your right heel, with your toes raised slightly, to your right.

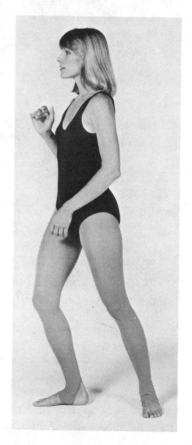

2. Now shift your weight to your right foot. Your left leg is relaxed.

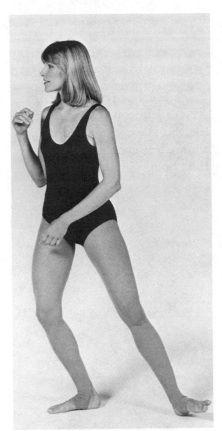

3. Step out with your left foot, with your heel touching the floor slightly.

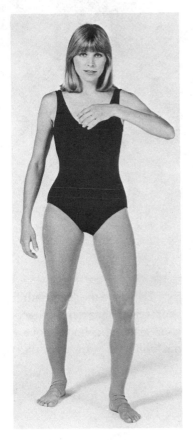

4. Shift your weight to your left foot and pivot to the front. As you do, your left arm rises, with the palm turned in, to chest height, while your right arm sinks gently to your side. Follow by pivoting slightly to the left and perform similar movements to "ward off with right hand."

Squatting Down

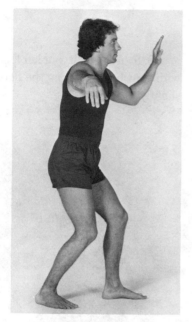

1. Stand with your body weight on your left foot, with your right leg relaxed and your left arm bent at the elbow and the palm of your hand facing outward.

2. Pivot to the right, shifting your weight onto your right foot; your arms and body move in one unit.

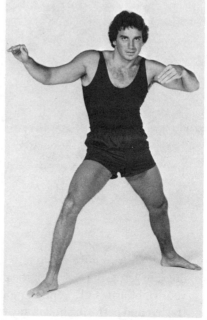

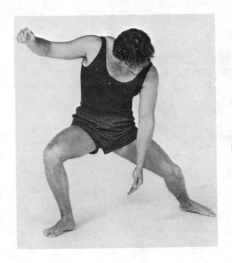

3. Squat down, your left arm dropping gently in front of you and your right arm extended with the wrist limp.

Golden Cock Stands on One Leg

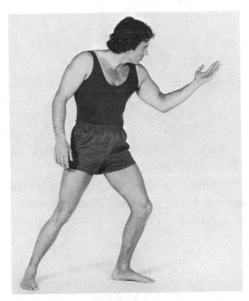

1. This posture follows "Squatting Down." From a squatting position, your weight shifts forward to your left foot and your body rises, with your left arm, slightly bent, extending.

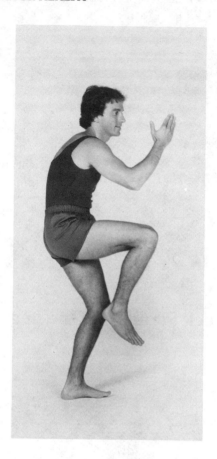

2. Lift your right knee to waist height; your right arm, with elbow bent, lifts upward in an arc, while your left arm falls to your side. Notice how your left knee is slightly curved.

Note: Don't raise your knee too high or you will begin to feel tension. Let your eyes follow your hand. And remember to move slowly!

Tae Kwon Do: Agility for Mind and Body

When Gus Hoefling, the trainer for the Philadelphia Phillies, wants to get his ballplayers in shape, he doesn't send them out to the playing field. Instead, he dons a *gi*—the pajamalike garb of the martial arts, and takes the team through strength and flexibility exercises. To Hoefling, the martial arts develop a keen sense of concentration, which has been key to Hoefling's work with various Phillies pitchers.

Similarly, when linebacker Andre Tippett wants to improve his flexibility and hone his speed, he turns to karate. Tippett feels his extensive training in the martial arts has given him a decisive edge on the football field, and the flexibility he's gained helps keep him free of injury as well. In fact, Tippett's use of karate in his training has been so successful that it's inspired many of his fellow New England Patriots to do the same.

Practicing the martial arts may not make you as successful as a professional baseball or football player in your training, but it can help. Used properly, this ancient art of self-defense can improve your flexibility, enhance concentration and fine-tune technique.

The realm of martial arts is so vast that you can select a form according to a specific physical trait or skill you want to develop—Okinawan karate for general upper-body strength, for example, or judo for grappling and wrestling techniques. Or, if you're interested in enhancing concentration, any of the many forms would do, since all require mental discipline.

We chose to highlight a form of karate known as Tae Kwon Do, because of its emphasis on strengthening the legs and improving overall flexibility. (Some words of caution, though. Tae Kwon Do is for those who are already in fairly good shape. Also, in order to get the most benefit from these exercises and perform them safely, it's best to do them under the guidance of an experienced instructor.) Since conditioning of the legs is important to any sport, and flexibility is a key to preventing injury, this martial art form is a good choice. Moreover, because this Korean form is popular in the United States, it is a practical choice should you decide to study the art further.

Warming Up

Before you try our four suggested techniques, warm up thoroughly with the following stretches, concentrating on your legs.

With your back leaning against a wall, lift and pull one leg toward your face. Do not bend your knee. Repeat with your other leg. Then repeat the stretch by raising your leg to the side. These will stretch your groin muscles and hamstrings and, to a lesser degree, your quadriceps.

To further stretch the groin area, do straddles and splits; ease yourself down. When doing the splits, be sure to alternate legs front and back.

Also try "butterflies." Sitting with your knees bent and the soles of your feet together, work your knees closer and closer to the floor.

Now sit in a straddle position and lean your chest toward your right knee, then toward a spot between your knees, then toward your left knee. This will stretch your hamstrings and your lower back.

Be sure to stretch the lower back fully during the appropriate exercises. Also, do some trunk twists, as demonstrated in chapter 8. These are important, since most of the power in Tae Kwon Do is generated from weight transfer and midbody twisting.

All the Right Moves

Once your muscles are warm and loose, you are ready to try our four suggested Tae Kwon Do moves for enhancing flexibility: the Roundhouse Kick, Punches, the Side Kick, and the Front Snap Kick.

Most of these exercises are similar in that they focus on the legs, but each is different in the precise way it stretches your muscles. And the benefits are likely to be more extensive than simply increased flexibility. Flexibility aids coordination, timing, speed and concentration. Weekend athletes who've taken up martial arts have been heard to rave about more specific benefits—from boosting batting averages (attributed to greater hip mobility) to relieving back pain.

According to football player Andre Tippett, the list is endless. "Even people in business could benefit from it. Work your 9:00 to 5:00, then go to the *dojo* (school) and work off your stress."

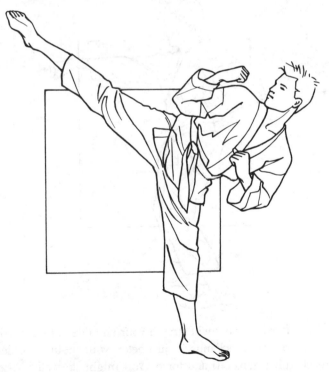

Roundhouse Kick. This will stretch your groin, ankle

extensors (because the ankle is cocked to deliver the kick with the ball of the foot), quadriceps, and hamstrings.

To execute the Roundhouse Kick:

1. Turn your left foot outward. It will serve as your base for this kick.
2. Lift your right foot, bending at the knee. This cocking, plus a slight shift of your body weight to the right, will allow maximum thrust.
3. Now shoot your foot straight in front of you, leading with the ball of the foot. Your foot and knee are at right angles to the floor.
4. Repeat, then do it with your other leg.

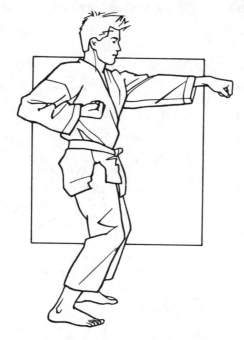

Punches.   These will stretch your shoulders, biceps, triceps, latissimus dorsi (the back muscles just below your shoulder blades—as you reach full extension) and torso. You might do well to use this upper-body exercise here, halfway through the series, since the others all emphasize your lower body, and your legs may become fatigued.

To execute the Punches:

1. Stand with your feet apart for balance.
2. Close your fingers into a fist. Keep one hand tucked chest-high near your body, the other extended, low and away from your body, for balance. In competition, the latter hand would be ready to block an opponent's blow.
3. Now, punch with the first hand, projecting straight out from its tucked position. Make this a quick motion. Snap your fist forward and feel the extension through the length of your arm.
4. Now bring that arm back into a tucked position and punch with your other hand.
5. Continue alternately.

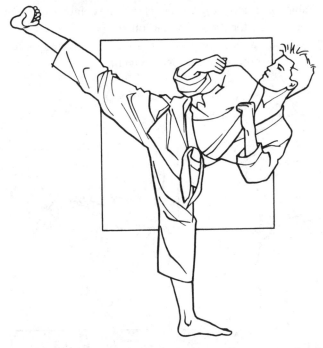

Side Kick.   The side kick will stretch the groin, the Achilles tendon (because of the way your ankle is cocked to deliver the kick), and the quadriceps and hamstrings as well. (In addition to being stretched in the delivery of the kick, these muscles will be twisted and stretched in the balancing leg.)

To execute the Side Kick:

1. Stand with your feet together. Your arms should be relaxed but ready at your sides for balance and, hypothetically, defense.
2. Lift one knee in front of you, balancing on the other foot. In effect, this move is the cocking of a trigger.
3. Swivel that same leg and hip and whip your leg to the side. (You may want to "walk" through this the first time, simply lifting your leg through the kick motion and touching it to a wall.) This imaginary blow should be sharply delivered with the heel and knife-edge of the foot.
4. Repeat, then try it with your other leg.

Slowly—over the course of days or even weeks, depending on how comfortable this is for you—try to increase the height and power of the kick. Do the same for the kicks that follow, too.

Always pick a target, even if it's just an imaginary spot in the air. This sharpens your concentration and technique.

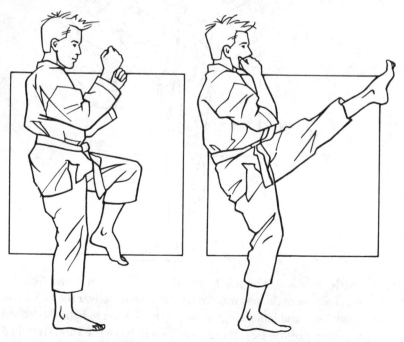

Front Snap Kick. This will stretch the groin, the ankle

extensors (because the toe is pointed while your foot's being raised), the quadriceps, and the hamstrings.

To execute the Front Snap Kick:

1. Stand with your feet slightly apart. Your hands should be ready at your sides, extended slightly for balance.
2. Begin by lifting your thigh, bend your knee, then gradually build momentum and snap your lower leg through the kick. Point the toe as you swing your foot upward, but then cock your ankle to strike with a flat foot.
3. Repeat, then do it with your other leg.

Don't Do
These Stretches

"Every week we see more injuries from stretching than injuries that are a result of stiffness," says Richard H. Dominguez, M.D., instructor of orthopedic surgery at Loyola University Medical Center. "People are no longer limiting themselves to that gentle, beneficial, natural stretching; now they are trying to become contortionists.

"Flexibility should not be a goal in itself but the result of muscle strengthening and training," he says. "A strengthening of the muscles around the joint naturally increases flexibility. If you can bend a joint beyond your ability to control it with muscle strength, you risk either tearing the muscles, tendons or ligaments that support the joint, or damaging the joint surface itself through abnormal pressure upon it.

"I see runners all the time who say, 'Boy, this running business has got my back sore.' And then you ask them what they've been doing, and they've been toe-touching and stretching prior to running. *People* magazine had a big story about Johnny Kelley, who's everybody's favorite marathoner. Well, what does he do to warm up? He heats himself a cup of coffee, then goes out and starts running," adds Dr. Dominguez.

The "old-fashioned way" for warming up is still Dr. Dominguez's recommendation: "Take a light jog until you work up a light sweat, then increase your activity."

"The Exercise Hit List"

Of all the stretches athletes perform, Dr. Dominguez has pinpointed eight for his "Exercise Hit List" of stretches that you shouldn't do. They are: Yoga Plow, Hurdler's Stretch, Duck Walk (and Deep Knee Bend), Stiff Leg Raise, Knee Stretch, Sit-Up, Toe Touch and Ballet Stretch. (EDITOR'S NOTE: Not all exercise physiologists agree with Dr. Dominguez. While people with unresolved low back pain or a history of back problems should avoid these stretches, others may be able to do them safely. If Dr. Dominguez's cautions apply to you, safe and healthful substitutes appear throughout this book.)

Why these eight?

"None of those exercises achieves what it is intended to do, number one," says Dr. Dominguez. "None of them is essential for high performance or just general fitness or even back strengthening. So you don't need to do any of them.

"And, number two, they will injure a number of people. Just because some people can do them and get away with it doesn't mean they're safe."

Here's "The Exercise Hit List" from Dr. Dominguez's book *Total Body Training* in somewhat more detail.

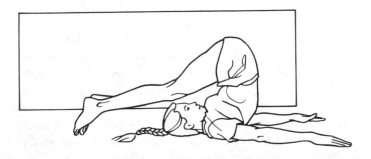

Yoga Plow. Holding your legs over your head while lying on your back carries with it a triple whammy: It is one of the few activities known to modern humanity in which you can injure your neck and back at the same time you're inducing a stroke. "The plow," explains Dr. Dominguez, "puts inordinate stretch and stress on the blood vessels to the brain and the upper spinal cord," effectively kinking the vertebral artery, cutting off circulation and potentially doing grievous damage. The Yoga Plow also places too much pressure on spinal disks and ligaments. And, last but not least, it can cause permanent fiber destruction in the cauda equina (the base of the spine) and the sciatic nerves by stretching nerve fibers beyond their length. "It's as though you are trying to pull out your nerves," says Dr. Dominguez. Enough said. Don't do it.

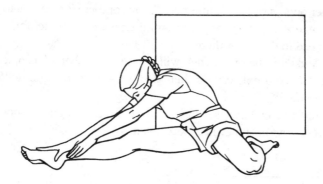

Hurdler's Stretch.   Extremely popular these days, this maneuver (which involves leaning forward and touching your feet alternately) stretches the muscles and ligaments in the groin farther than the Master Planner's blueprint designed them to go. Chronic groin pull is the classic, painful result. Moreover, it wreaks havoc on your knees, leading to injury of the meniscus cartilage (which attaches directly to the shin bone) and, even worse, to a steady, long-term taffy-pull of the medial collateral ligament, the one that helps stabilize the knee. Say goodbye to the meniscus and medial collateral—say hello to surgery. The sciatic nerve also gets a flogging, especially in older athletes.

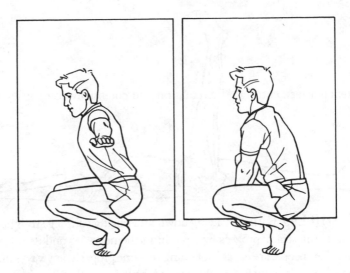

Duck Walk (and Deep Knee Bend). Dr. Dominguez points out that squatting down to walk like a duck in a deep-knee position was the first exercise ever to be condemned by the President's Council on Physical Fitness. Do it one time too many and you'll find yourself writhing on the floor, quacking rather loudly for help for your torn lateral (knee) cartilage.

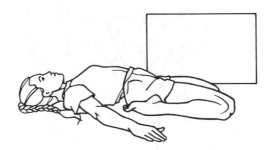

Knee Stretch. Tucking your legs under your buttocks and leaning backward is also harmful, according to Dr. Dominguez."If you look at the angle of the lower leg," says Dr. Dominguez, "you see that it clearly exceeds the actual skeletal range of motion of the knee." This does a great deal more harm than good—if it does any good at all. The patellar and collateral knee ligaments get stretched and strained, destabilizing the knees.

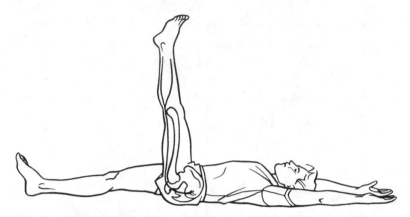

Stiff Leg Raise.   Lying down and raising your leg straight up subverts the sciatic process by stretching the nerve beyond its normal limits. Few people are capable of doing this one properly, anyway—most can't keep their spine flat on the ground, a weakness that leads to lower back pressure on the ligaments, muscles and disks. So why do it?

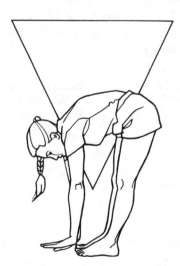

Toe Touch.   Most of us have been doing this one—bending down to touch our toes from a standing position—practically since kindergarten. According to Dr. Dominguez, swooping forward to plant your palms firmly on the floor does a good job of zapping the posterior longitudinal ligament, which is one of the main supporting ligaments in the spine. It can also undo a disk. "The muscles of the back cannot give any support when you are toe-touching," explains Dr. Dominguez. "You are actually stretching and hanging by your ligaments." The poor, beleaguered sciatic nerve risks being yanked from its connections, too. Dr. Dominguez thinks that most runners with back pain owe it all to the Toe Touch—which doesn't relax a tight back but actually makes the muscles tighter—and to the Hurdler's Stretch. (For a safer alternative to the Toe Touch, see the Floor Touch, in chapter 8.)

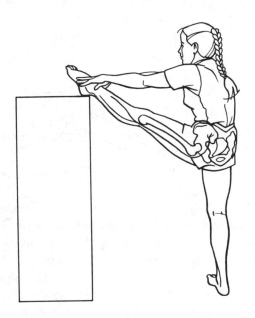

Ballet Stretch.   Raising your leg and resting it well above the level of your hip on a barre is a good way to put your tutu in a sling. Sharp zings down the legs from unnaturally elongated sciatic nerves accompany risky stretches of the back of the knee, low-back ligaments, muscles, joints and disks. This exercise was designed for dancers willing to pay the price in order to achieve their art's "abnormal, injury-producing postures." Unless you're waiting for a callback from the Bolshoi, skip it.

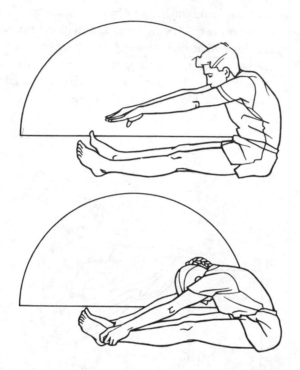

Sit-Up. The type of Sit-Ups that require you to bend from the waist with your legs extended straight in front of you is one of the traditional Dynamic Duo, with push-ups being the other. Sit-Ups are practically an All-American institution, a holy item, and criticism of them as hazardous comes awfully close to phys-ed sacrilege. Meet Dr. Richard Dominguez, heretic: "The goal of Sit-Ups is to strengthen the abdominal muscles. But after you come up about 30 degrees, you maximally shorten your abdominals. Then you're doing a hip exercise. It just doesn't tighten up your belly. It doesn't flatten your abdomen at all." Besides, he says, to sit up with momentum and pass the upright or gravity-neutral position results in back strain and nerve elongation. Much better is the Bent-Knee Sit-Up. It relaxes the sciatic nerve, which is, as we've seen, ground zero for so many of the stretching exercises. But if you have back trouble, even Bent-Knee Sit-Ups ought to be avoided.